ADDICTION AND MENTAL HEALTH

LEARN HOW SUBSTANCE ABUSE AND MENTAL ILLNESS OFTEN GO TOGETHER

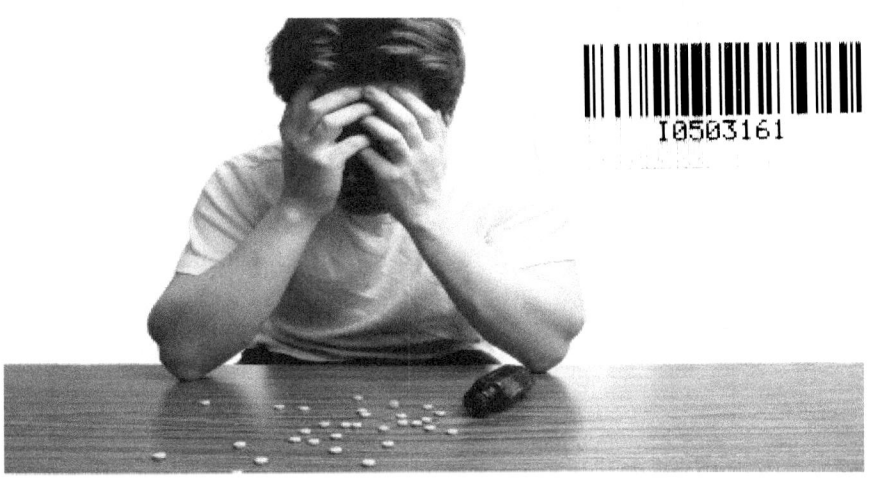

I0503161

By Patricia A Carlisle

Introduction

I want to thank you and congratulate you for choosing the book, *"ADDICTION AND MENTAL HEALTH: Learn how Substance Abuse and Mental Illness often go together"*.

This book contains proven steps and strategies on how substance abuse and mental illness often go together.

Addiction and mental health is a serious and critical issue in our society. Imagine a city occupied by drug addicts and mentally ill individuals, how do you think such a city can fair? Probably you would agree that such a place is actually building a foundation set on a time bomb. When a person is addicted to a substance which serves a specific purpose and on the long run, the addiction becomes abusive; there is every tendency that such person can become a dangerous member of society. Hence, the problem of substance abuse; is a topic that links up with mental illness and often go together in many instances.

The fact remains that, some people are having issues of abuse of substance which resulted into mental health problems while some experience mental health conditions as a result of the fact that they probably were born that way or that they were exposed to certain conditions that led them to the problem. It is also on record that; it is either a person is suffering from one of the two or both.

However, mental health problems are often interwoven and ascribe to substance abuse by the common man and that one of them is more vulnerable and definitely lead to the other. But experts have been able to analyze the difference between the two and the functionality of the two is going to be determined in this book

Thanks again for choosing this book, I hope you enjoy it!

The information herein is offered for informational purposes solely, and is universal as so. The presentation of the information is without contract or any type of guarantee assurance.

The trademarks that are used are without any consent, and the publication of the trademark is without permission or backing by the trademark owner. All trademarks and brands within this book are for clarifying purposes only and are the owned by the owners themselves, not affiliated with this document.

Patricia A. Carlisle, MSW, CBT

Patricia Carlisle- A Master Social Worker and a Cognitive Behavioral Therapist (CBT) gives out an expression of how important it is for an individual to take into consideration the concept of self-assessment to know what human, technical and conceptual skills they posses to perform or to achieve what they desire, or to deal with everyday life. However, every particular group of people has their own unique set of ideas, traditions and events including the frame of mind according to which people perform but there are many who faces problems and fail to maintain a healthy mind set affecting their behaviors and performance to those around them.

People like Patricia Carlisle are among those who have felt this urge of serving people and helping them out of their mental crisis towards a healthy life. She has experienced some close encounters in her personal life regarding mental health issues in her family and friends that has encouraged her to pursue this as her career.

Currently Patricia Carlisle is serving as a Certified On-Line Cognitive Behavioral Therapist with an extensive 15years of experience using Cognitive-Behavior Therapy Techniques. She envisions a world where everyone gets mental health treatment with no mental health stigma and to make it real she has already set up her own Holistic Measure Online Comprehensive Behavioral Healthcare Company after retiring from The Nord Center in The Partial Hospitalization Program (PHP) Dept for 5 years and Murtis H. Taylor Mental Health Center as a mental health counselor, psychological support technician and case manager for 10 years to emulsify her skills more professionally. Along with this, she has wrote down her passion as a clinician in 25 or more short books to help individuals and families get their life back, freeing them of the restraints of negative thinking, anxiety and depression by using different approaches. She is highly appreciated among her clients for her flexibility and professionalism of dealing with them graciously.

To reach her, make use of her direct website address: http://therapist2013.wix.com/e-therapy . As she is ready to inspire hope and contribute to health and well-being by providing the best online health care through comprehensive practice, education and research.

TABLE OF CONTENT

Conclusion

Preview Of 'ADDICTION: LEARN HOW TO BREAK ANY ADDICTION'

Chapter 1

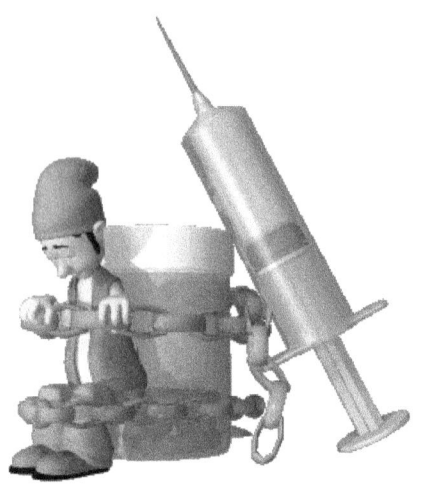

SUBSTANCE ABUSE MAY NOT BE A LEAD CAUSE OF MENTAL ILLNESS

If we want to generally view the issue, we can bring out some salient points that will definitely move us to draw inferences where substance abuse may not necessary be the lead cause of mental illness in some cases. Doctors in the field of medical research have given a detailed analysis of their experiences with various patients in the hospital, these patients also come from all works of life and at some point suffered from several combining factors which are inclusive of substance abuse and naturally occurring mentally driven health problems that developed exclusively as a result of change in circumstances or some form of environmental factors.

The fact remains that, some people are having issues of abuse of substance which resulted into mental health problems while some experience mental health conditions as a result of the fact that they probably were born that way or that they were exposed to certain conditions that led them to the problem. It is also on record that; it is either a person is suffering from one of the two or both. However, mental health problems are often interwoven and ascribe to substance abuse by the common man and that one of them is more vulnerable and definitely lead to the other. But, experts have been able to analyze the difference between the two and the functionality of the two is going to be determined in this book.

At least two in every ten adult are suffering from a condition of diagnosable mental problem or disorders a result of various substance usages and other factors responsible for mental problem according to the National Institute of Mental Health. When any one of the factors responsible for mental health problem is caused as a result of naturally occurring syndrome such as a genetic or biological vulnerability, then if there is any attempt or venture into the use of substance abuse no matter the minute or magnitude of the usage of such substance either small or big, there is the potential and high risk that such usage will further worsen or increase the gravity of the mental health problem.

That is one of the consequences of substance abuse by a person naturally having traces of mental health problem. The substance may not necessary be causing the mental health problem, but, it will definitely invoke a factor that can trigger up a mental health illness that will begin to show some symptoms. Many people have these characteristics inherent in them without them knowing that they have this problem.

The enabling factor is the driving power of addiction, so when addiction first becomes a problem to an individual the mental health problem begins to creep in until diagnoses. Hence, it is this dual nature of mental health problems that constitute the propositions that has been bringing into limelight a detailed uncomplicated explanation of the various forms of mental illness causes addictions, substance abuse and natural re-occurring factor which is responsible for mental disorders or poor health.

Chapter 2

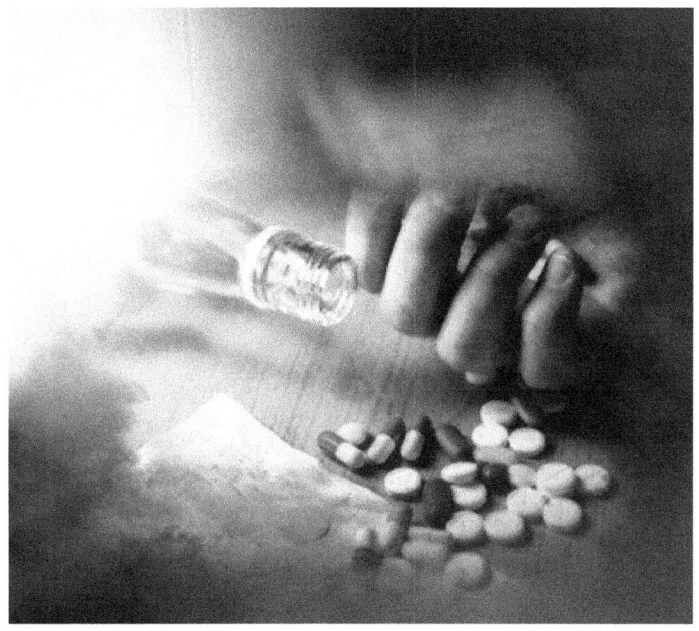

THE RELATION BETWEEN SUBSTANCE ABUSE AND MENTAL ILLNESS

The complications of mental illness are further compounded by abuses from drugs and alcoholism, causing and posing a big challenge to acquire the proper and adequate diagnosis that will bring lasting solution to the problem.

Illness as a result of mental problem associated with addiction to alcohol or drug abuse are interwoven in a string of complex undertone. The problem associated with this type of relationship is as a result of self-medication in most cases where drugs are administered by an individual on himself without following the right prescriptions and also without seeking medical attention from a licensed medical practitioner. While the person engages in self medication, there is every tendency that when the individual gets the requisite temporary relief from self medication, he or she will always revisit the drugs and also may continue subsequent intake to an extent that will medically exceed the requisite dosage.

Same also can be said of Alcoholism. When a person is addicted to alcohol, the person no longer drinks alcohol socially, he or she takes it as if their whole life depends on it and when it gets to that level the addition has culminated into a abuse and the substance will definitely affect not only the mental stability but also it will push to other consequences of mental illnesses, dullness, sleeping off while on duty and risking accident while driving and so many other common incidental occurrences resulting from abuse of substance as it relates to mental illness.

Always note that one particular disorder can be very worse than the other. The person who takes hard drugs may be more violent than a person who takes excessive alcohol. Alcohol often lead to depression and inability to think straight and do that right thing at the right time while drugs can become very detrimental to mental stability more deeper than alcohol.

Drugs like cocaine, opium and other drugs like them are capable of destroying the brain cells. A documentary presented by James Garbutt; stated "Mental illnesses can increase the risk for alcoholism or drug abuse, sometimes because of self induced medicating and meanwhile it is to be noted that alcoholism can lead to significant anxiety and depression which may be indistinguishable from a mental illness. Finally, one disorder can be worse than the other." James Garbutt is a professor of psychiatry at the University of North Caroline, USA.

Therefore, we can deduce from available facts on medical records that drugs and alcoholism addiction resulting from abuse of both substances and other psychiatric problems or disorders are sometimes simultaneously occurring together at the same time. Meanwhile, the two are the distinct anomalies that should be treated as such in order to achieve a problem solved or healing outcome for affected persons.

Chapter 3

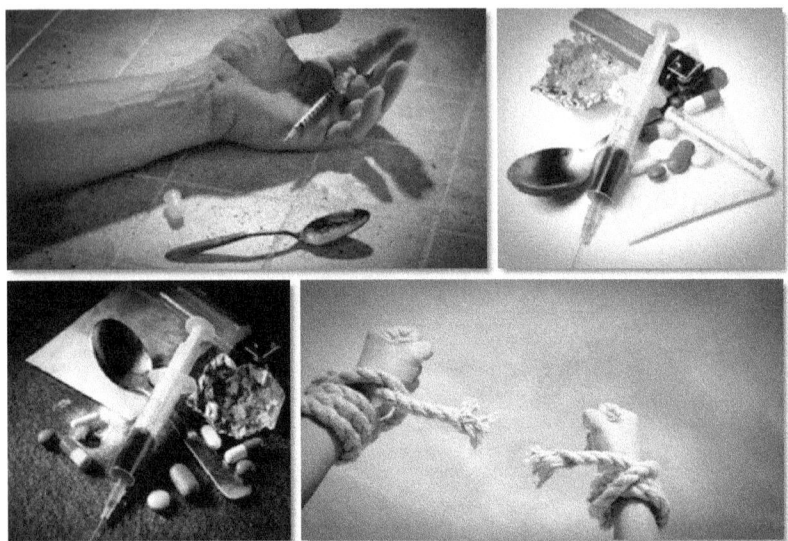

ABUSE OF DRUGS AND MENTAL ILLNESS CONDITION

Bipolar disorder: commonly referred to as mood swings is one of the common characteristics of drug abused person who suffer mental illness. Here we see how substance abuse based on drug usage affects the mood or lead to mood swings, it can be for a very bad mood when this happens. Then consequences is pushing moods of the individuals towards a deteriorating positions that can make the person to become helpless such as tilting the moods towards violence, ecstasy, or even criminally motivated moods that is common among hard drug users. Hence, abuse of substances and mental illness always go together when it comes to this headline, because majority of those who are having mental rehabilitation in psychiatric hospital sections that has to do with people having problems of drug addictions are prominent in that section of the psychiatric hospital.

Some notable celebrities and sports men and women also have had several cases of drug abuse which ruined many of these famous people careers. Some have been able to recover from it while others have yet to get over it. So in this aspect there is a close link between abuse of substance and mental illness.

Chapter 4

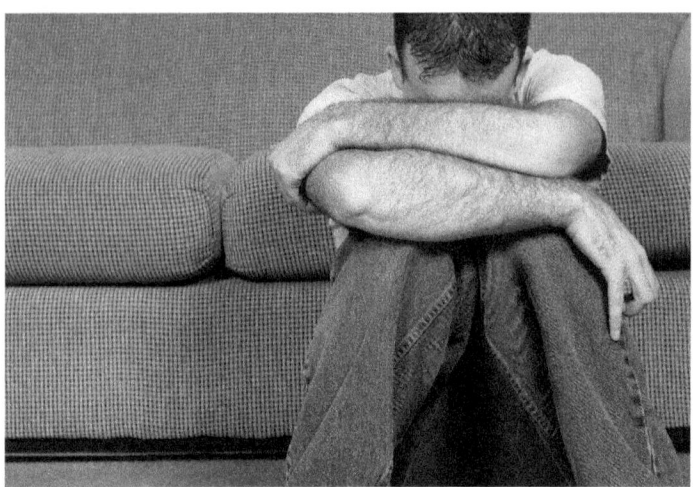

HOW DRUGS CAUSE ANXIETY DISORDERS

Recent studies have shown that excessive alcoholism has also lead to depression of people who are addicted to it causing them to pass through difficulties associated with emotional problems, anxieties and depression disorders.

While being stress up, what readily comes to the mind of alcohol addiction prone individuals is to take the substance to get relief and what they end up achieving are further anxiety and more depression resulting from the effects of excessive alcoholism. Some heartbroken person often results to alcoholism, leaving a terrible influence and control by the liquor. Quite often actions carried out by a drunken man or woman is that they may not be controlled by the senses, and this can be dangerous. In some jurisdictions, mere taking of alcohol is not a defense for committing a crime, in actual fact, being drunk can be a criminal offence in many jurisdictions. So alcohol prone persons are liable to commit crime.

Psychotic phenomenon commonly referred to as schizophrenia is a common problem with people who are affected by substance abuse and mental illness, here we make reference to delusions and hallucinations which will always resort to abuse of substance and this may further lead to further mental illness, so both go together and work hand in hand to cause mental illness because the substance abuse will be an option for a person that is suffering from psychotic problems

Chapter 5

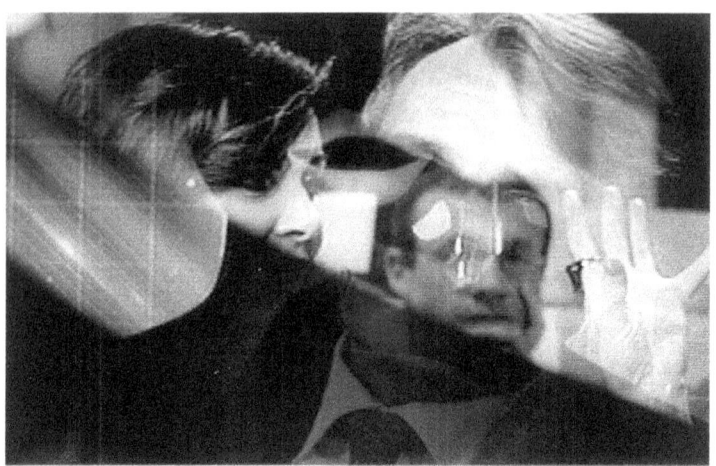

IMPAIRED MENTAL JUDGMENT

When there is substance abuse, there is the likelihood of impairment of mental judgment. You will always have instances of having to deal with sound judgment or making a decision without any influence from drugs or alcohol.

Naturally, when a person is acting normal without any influence, the problem of mental illness does not arise. But when substances abuse is involved, there is definitely the propensity to act adversely contrary to the requisite norms and practices in the society.

That means that; when substance abuse is involved and the senses cannot be able to act or think rightly then we can conclude that there is direct link or that substance abuse and mental illness goes together. Persons with proven mental disorders also have the propensity to take or consume the highest quantity of drugs or alcohol. This is a very dangerous situation if it is experience among persons in any society.

Chapter 6

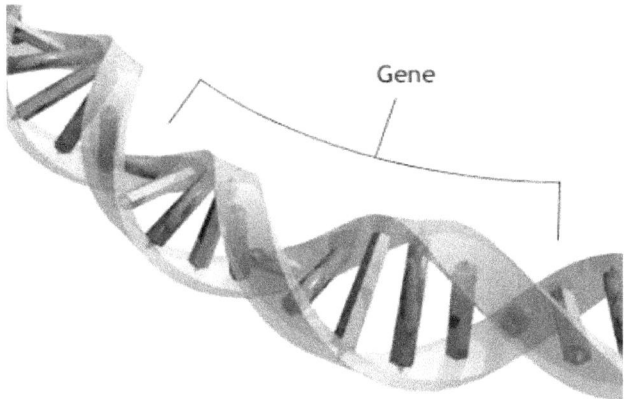

GENETIC FACTORS

When couples get married, one thing is certain, that it is naturally expected that the union will breed children. Healthy offspring are expected from healthy marriages. But there are some natural selections that take place during the process of procreation, the children of such marriage will probably inherit from their parents certain genes and characteristics associated with inheritance. Yes! Inheritable traits and genes present in the parents will be transferred to the offspring of the family, at least one among four children from a couple will inherit some behavior or characteristics common to both or one of the parents and when the genes are transferred to a child, and the child while growing up to become an adult exposes himself or herself to a condition that will trigger substance abuse that can lead to mental illness, then that situation proves that the parents played a big role in transmitting the problem along their lineage.

Hence, the study of genetics has proven so many times that genes are transmitted from parents to their offspring and sometimes disorders can be discovered in children from families who have a medical history of mental illness. The environment where a child is developing will definitely help a child to grow properly and help assist in suppressing situations that can cause mental illness to prop up. But that is if the surrounding environment is conducive for proper development.

Chapter 7

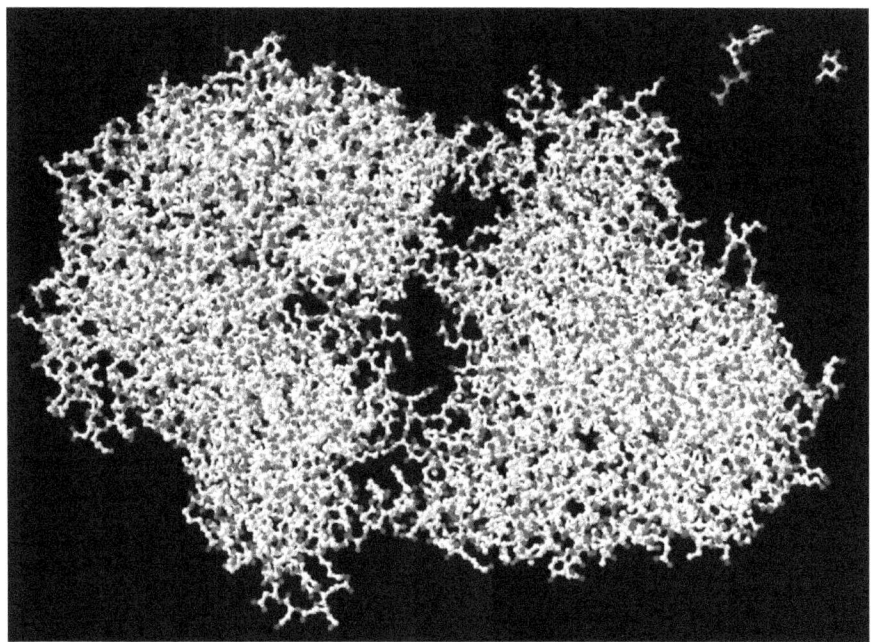

CHEMICAL DEFICIENCY

The human body is found to have certain body metabolism that would enable a balanced and composition of the body structure "chemical wise"-neuro-chemical essentials made up of strands and threads in the human nervous system linking to the brain and an imbalance can cause serious mental disorders due to impeding factors such as addiction taking place can result to serious mental problems altogether.

For instance, when the amount of (serotonin) which is a chemical substance responsible to the functioning of the brains is seriously affected by excessive alcohol addiction and also disordered anxiety disorders occurring many times. It will lead to mental disorders common to the malfunctioning of a system of brain chemical medically referred to as monoamine exidases.

These chemical once it is affected by addiction, it will be tilted in its content and this affect the brains cells and that can spell trouble to the addicted individual who is always depending on substance which he is already abusing while using it. Hence, abuse of substance and mental illness goes together in this instant.

Chapter 8

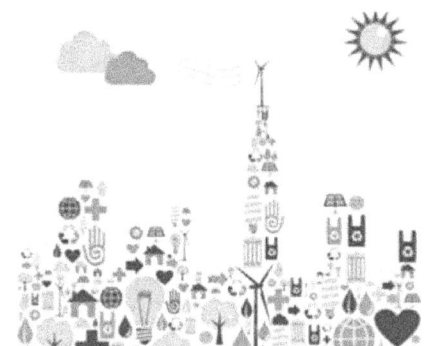

Environment and health

SHARED ENVIRONMENT

Have you ever thought about the environment, how the environment gets polluted? When you visualize polluted environment, what do you see? Can you see destruction, dirty and filthy environment? Can you imagine the disease that can plague people living around such an environment?

Such can also be linked to a place where we have people being influence by drug addiction and abuse of substances that lead to mental illness. The negative influence from such environment can be seen to affect people from areas like slumps, ghetto and suburbs were streets gangs are usually found doing drugs, places around the world where these slumps are found are prone to criminal activities and worst of it is that these kind of places are always found with beehives of activities from drug addicts.

Chapter 9

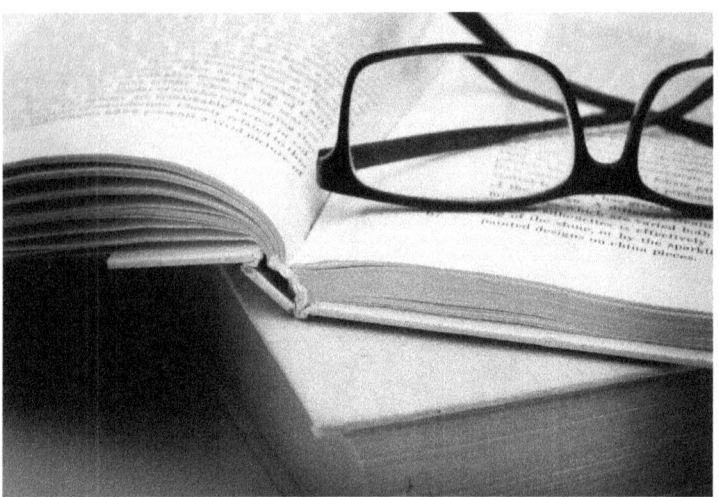

WHAT IS IMPORTANT TO UNDERSTAND

with the limitations to this statements being exceptional cases of genetic and inherited naturally proven problems associated with mental illness resulting from heredity. many instance of self inflicted abuse resulting from usage of drug addiction or alcoholism that lead to mental illness are also abound. so with the detailed explanation as enumerated above we can deduce the extent at which substance abuse plays a part in mental illness.

Without influence from drugs or alcohol also have the tendencies to make substance abuse case, a worst thing that can further aggravate the problem the person is having. Some people with the problem often sometimes experience deplorable situation of mental illness associated with a psychiatric disorder deeper than just influence from substance abuse. This kind of problem needs more critical and intensive care and treatment.

There are also those who have post traumatic mental conditions and may however recover from mental illness, there may not be as a result of usage of substance but resulting from stress disorders, personality or characterized disorders, antisocial, personality disorders or empathy inability, sleep disorders, post medical treatment/rehabilitation circumstances that may cause changes in psychological trauma.   It is also important to understand that some of the mental illness resulting from substance addiction which symptoms are addictive or psychiatric in nature are very hard to control or stopped and it is often difficult to distinguish which symptoms are psychiatric and which is addictive.

In other words an individual with the problem of mental illness would need to stay clear from any substance for a period not less than two weeks in order to be able to study and determine the properties or the real symptoms to be treated. Although both substance abuse and addiction are capable of a bipolar disorder manifestation; some level of knowledge about treatment is also required to be able to contain the problem. However, some professionals would suggest that both can be treated concurrently, it is also possible to totally eliminate one symptom while we continue to battle the order till the problems finally abates.

Conclusion

Thank you again for choosing this book!

Many people today have the misconception and often times usually equate mental illness to substance abuse only. This is not always the cases in most cases we have seen instances where genetic factors, environment and post traumatic conditions also affect mental illness. The fact still remains certain that substance abuse plays a very huge role among the many factors responsible for the mental illness and the twosome goes together.

Parents are advised to take control of the development of their children and area very seriously because the majority of the youths are involved in one problems or the other that has to do with mental stability due to influence from peer group to do drugs; the most common type of mental illness threat factor. These kids are being lured into doing drugs and before you know it, they end up having serious mental illness issues.

Parents can go for counseling in the area of mental illness for help with early detection and also always examine and monitor the activities of your kids, reading e-books like this one that will enlighten them on the salient issues pertaining to various topics that are linked to proper development of your children and entire family. The best bet is to stick to this advice and avoid the risk of having to deal with huge medical bills or even losing your young ones to unhealthy metal illness caused by substance abuse.

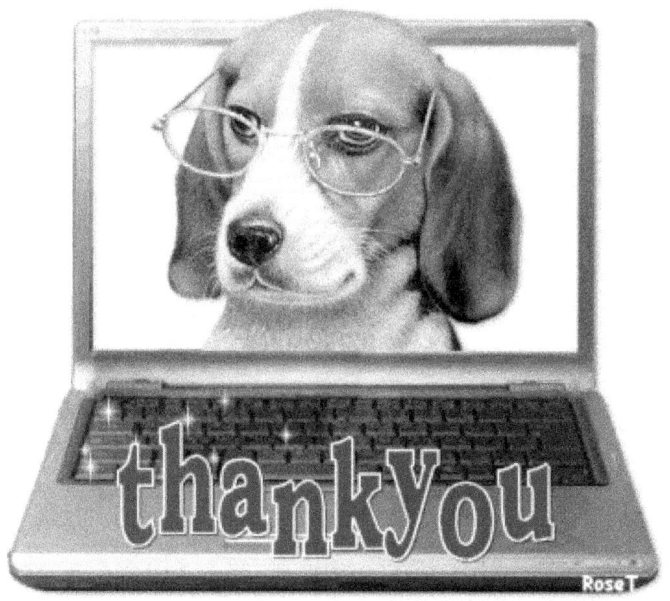

Finally, if you enjoyed this book, would you be kind enough to leave a review for this book on Amazon? It'd be greatly appreciated!

Thank you and good luck!

Preview Of 'ADDICTION: LEARN HOW TO BREAK ANY ADDICTION'

Chapter 1

CAUSES OF ADDICTION

There are several reasons why addiction is very frightening. The term "addiction" originates from a Latin word referred to as "enslaved by". So from this meaning, we can see that a person suffering from addiction actually lacks control over what he or she is addicted to and this is why many people who are addicted to drugs or some other things as discussed earlier are having a hard time quitting it and have their lives destroyed by it.

Addiction causes a very strong influence and distortion on the brain in different ways which can be categorized or grouped into 3 different categories which are one, a very strong desire for the object, two losing control over the usage of such object and three a continuous usage regardless of the harmful adverse effects of its usage. It was formerly, especially some years ago that experts tend to equate substances like alcohol and hard drugs or narcotics to be the only source responsible for addiction.

However, it has been discovered by scientist in the world of technology that it is not only continuous usage of hard drugs or drinking of alcohol alone that is responsible for addiction. Neuro-imaging technologies has also indicated that some pleasures like shopping, gambling, sex or pornography and sporting activities can also influence the human brain in a very strong manner to the extent that addiction begins to develop. Actually, addiction is not an inborn behavior; hence, no one is an "addictionist" so to say. But, people get entangled into it because of what they come across in life which gradually becomes pleasurable to them.

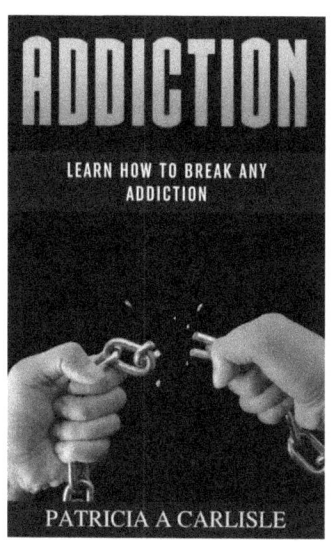

Go to Amazon.com to finish reading about ADDICTION: Learn How to Break Any Addiction.

Check Out My Other Books

Below you'll find some of my other popular books that are popular on Amazon and Kindle as well. Alternatively, you can visit my author page on Amazon to see other work done by me. (https://amazon.com/author/patriciacarlisle)

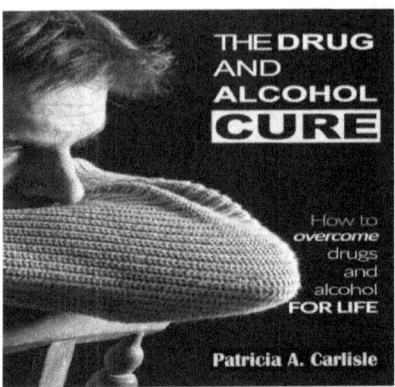

The DRUG and ALCOHOL Cure: How to overcome drugs and alcohol for life.

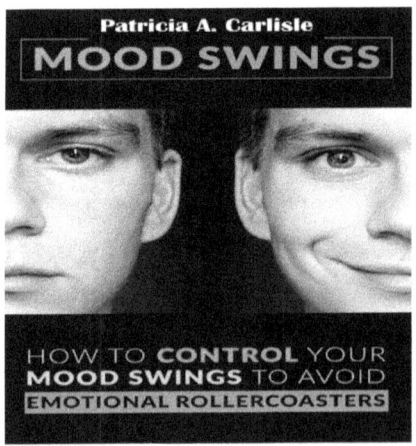

MOOD SWINGS: How To control Your Mood Swings to Avoid Emotional Rollercoaster's.

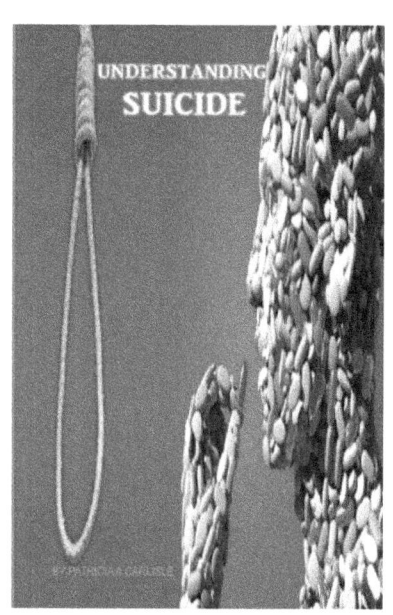

UNDERSTANDING SUICIDE.

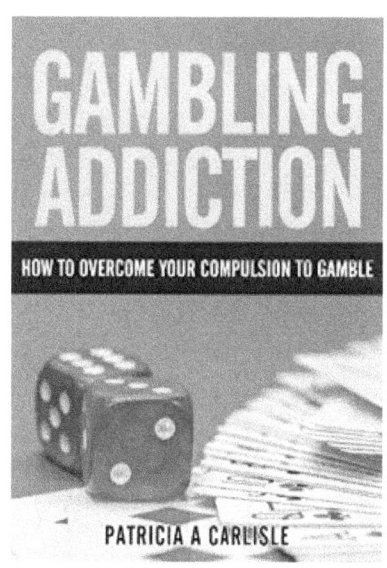

**GAMBLING ADDICTION: HOW TO OVERCOME
YOUR COMPULSION TO GAMBLE.**

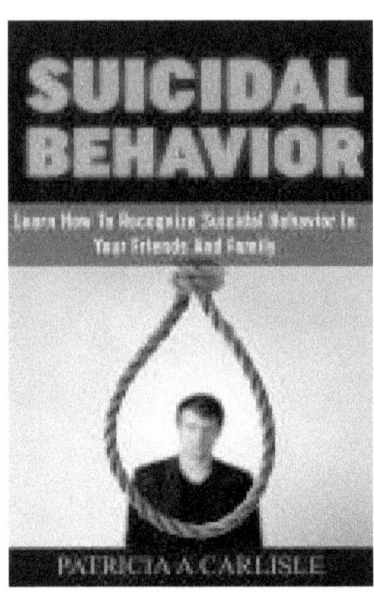

SUICIDAL BEHAVIOR: LEARN HOW TO RECOGNIZE SUICIDAL BEHAVIOR IN YOUR FRIENDS AND FAMILY.

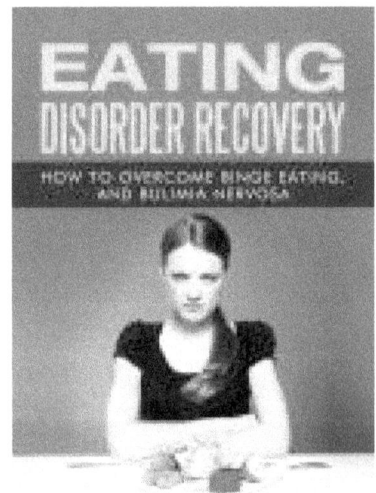

EATING DISORDER RECOVERY: HOW TO OVERCOME BINGE EATING AND BULIMIA NERVOSA.

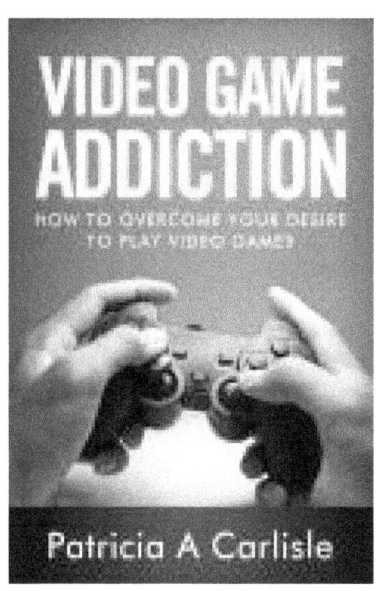

VIDEO GAME ADDICTION: HOW TO OVERCOME YOUR DESIRE TO PLAY VIDEO GAMES.

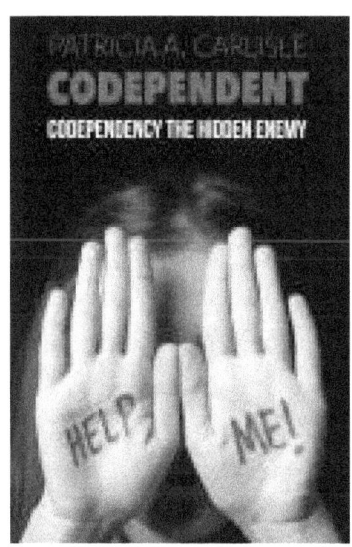

CODEPENDENT: CODEPENDENCY THE HIDDEN ENEMY.

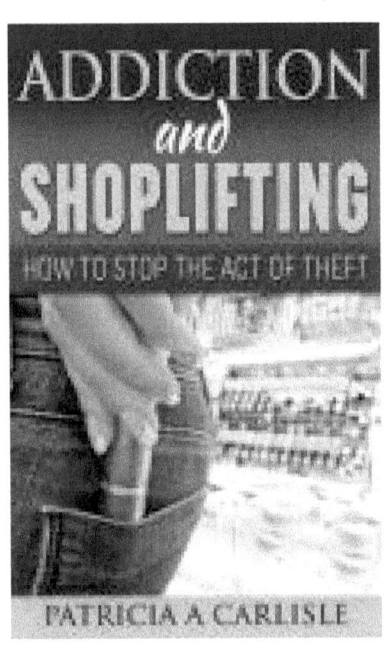

ADDICTION AND SHOPLIFTING: HOW TO STOP THE ACT OF THEFT.

You can simply search for these titles on the Amazon website to find them.

BONUS: SUBSCRIBE TO THE FREE BOOK

Beginners Guide to Yoga & Meditation

"Stressed out? Do You Feel Like The World Is Crashing Down Around You? Want To Take A Vacation That Will Relax Your Mind, Body And Spirit? Well this Easy To Read Step By Step

E-Book Makes It All Possible!"

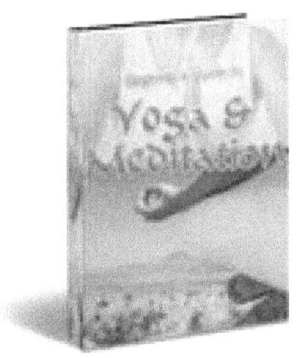

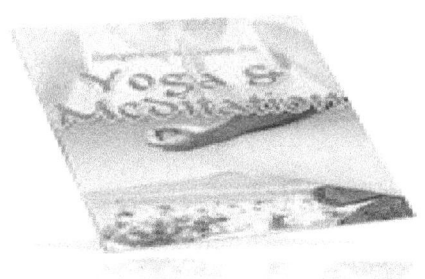

Instructions on how to join our mailing list, and receive a free copy of "Yoga and Meditation" can be found in any of my Kindle eBooks.

NOTES

NOTES

NOTES